Breast Cancer:

A Comprehensive Guide for Patients and Caregivers

By

Dr Steven R. Crews

Copyright © by Dr Steven R. Crews 2022.

Disclaimer

This book is not intended to replace your personal physician clinical advice and treatment or to provide counseling, therapy or treatment. Readers are strongly advised to consult their own qualified physicians regarding medical issues. By continuing to read this book, the reader agrees and acknowledges that neither the publisher nor the author is responsible for any losses, whether direct or indirect, that are incurred as a result of the application of information in this book. This includes, but it is not limited to, omissions, inaccuracies or errors .

Table of Contents

Introduction

Definition and Overview

Cancer of the breast is a type of cancer that develops in the cells of the breast and progresses to other parts of the body. It is more common in women, but it can occur in men as well. The most common type of breast cancer is ductal carcinoma, which starts in the cells that line the milk ducts of the breast.

Breast cancer can be benign (not cancerous) or malignant (cancerous). Benign breast tumors do not spread to other parts of the body and are not life-threatening. Malignant breast tumors, on the other hand, can spread to other parts of the body through the bloodstream or lymphatic system, and can be life-threatening if not treated.

Breast cancer can occur in different parts of the breast, including the ducts, lobules, and fatty and connective tissue. It can also spread to other parts of the body, such as the lymph nodes, bones, liver, and lungs.

Treatment for breast cancer may include surgery, chemotherapy, radiation therapy, hormonal therapy, or targeted therapy. The type of treatment depends on the stage and grade of the cancer, as well as the patient's age, overall health, and personal preferences. Early detection and diagnosis are key to improving the chances of successful treatment and survival.

Risk Factors and Causes

There are several risk factors and potential causes of breast cancer, including:

1.Gender: Breast cancer is much more common in women than in men, although men can also develop breast cancer.

2.Age: The risk of breast cancer increases with age, with the majority of cases occurring in women over the age of 50.

3.Family history: Having a family history of breast cancer, particularly a mother or sister with the disease, can increase your risk of developing breast cancer.

4.Genetic factors: Certain genetic mutations, such as BRCA1 and BRCA2, can increase the risk of breast cancer.

5.Personal history: Women who have previously had breast cancer are at an increased risk of developing the disease again.

6.Reproductive and menstrual history: Women who have their first menstrual period before the age of 12, go through menopause after the age of 55, have never given birth, or have a late age at first pregnancy may be at an increased risk of breast cancer.

7.Lifestyle factors: Alcohol consumption, obesity, and lack of physical activity may increase the risk of breast cancer.

8.Environmental and occupational exposures: Some studies have suggested that exposure to certain chemicals and radiation may increase the risk of breast cancer.

9.Hormone therapy: Long-term use of hormone therapy, particularly combination hormone therapy, may increase the risk of breast cancer.

It's important to note that having one or more of these risk factors does not necessarily mean that a person will develop breast cancer. It's also important to remember that many cases of breast cancer occur in people without any known risk factors.

Incidence and Prevalence

Breast cancer is a common type of cancer in women and, less commonly, in men. According to the World Health Organization (WHO), breast cancer is the most common cancer among women worldwide, accounting for 16% of all female cancers. In addition to this, among female patients, it is the second most common type of cancer that ultimately results in death, after only lung cancer.

The incidence of breast cancer refers to the number of new cases of breast cancer that are diagnosed in a population over a certain period of time. The prevalence of breast cancer refers to the total number of people living with breast cancer at a given time, including those who have been diagnosed with the disease and those who are in remission.

The incidence of breast cancer varies by age, with the risk of developing breast cancer increasing as a person gets older. In the United States, the average age at diagnosis is 61 years. The incidence of breast cancer is also higher in developed countries compared to developing countries, and it is more common in white women than in women of other racial and ethnic groups.

There are several factors that can increase the risk of developing breast cancer, including:

1.Age: The risk of breast cancer increases with age, with most cases occurring in women over the age of 50.

2.Family history: A person is more likely to develop breast cancer if they have a family history of the disease, especially if a close relative (such as a mother, sister, or aunt) has had breast cancer.

3.Genetics: Certain genetic mutations, such as BRCA1 and BRCA2, can increase the risk of breast cancer.

4.Hormones: Estrogen and progesterone, two hormones produced by the ovaries, can stimulate the growth of breast cancer cells. Women who have a longer exposure to these hormones, such as those who began menstruating at an early age or went through menopause at a later age, have a higher risk of breast cancer.

5.Lifestyle: Certain lifestyle factors, such as alcohol consumption, being overweight or obese, and not getting enough physical activity, have been linked to an increased risk of breast cancer.

There are several ways to reduce the risk of breast cancer, including:

1.Maintaining a healthy weight: Being overweight or obese can increase the risk of breast cancer, especially after menopause. A healthy weight can be maintained through diet and regular exercise, which can help minimize the risk.

2.Limiting alcohol consumption: Drinking alcohol, especially in large amounts, has been linked to an increased risk of breast cancer. Limiting alcohol consumption to no more than one drink per day for women and two drinks per day for men can help reduce the risk.

3.Getting regular physical activity: Being physically active can help reduce the risk of breast cancer. Aim for at least 150 minutes of moderate-intensity or 75 minutes of vigorous-intensity physical activity per week.

4.Breastfeeding: Breastfeeding can help reduce the risk of breast cancer, especially if it is done for a year or more.

5.Avoiding hormone therapy: Hormone therapy, which is often used to treat menopausal symptoms, has been linked to an increased risk of breast cancer. Avoiding hormone therapy or using the lowest effective dose for the shortest amount of time can help reduce the risk.

It is important to note that the risk of breast cancer can never be completely eliminated. However, making lifestyle changes and following recommended screening guidelines can help reduce the risk and improve the chances of detecting breast cancer early, when it is most treatable.

Symptoms and Diagnosis

Common Symptoms

The early stages of breast cancer may not cause any symptoms, so it is important to get regular mammograms and breast exams to detect it early. However, as the cancer progresses, it may cause the following symptoms:

1.A new lump or mass in the breast: A breast cancer tumor may feel hard, uneven, or lumpy, and may be painful to the touch.

2.Changes in the breast size or shape: The breast may feel swollen, look red or inflamed, or appear to be larger or shrinks.

3.Changes in the skin of the breast: The skin of the breast may look red, scaly, or thickened, or may have a rash or dimples.

4.Nipple changes: The nipple may become inverted, turn outward, or have discharge.

5.Swelling in the armpit: A cancerous tumor in the breast can cause swelling in the armpit or lymph nodes in the neck or collarbone.

It is important to note that these symptoms can also be caused by other conditions, such as an infection or benign breast tissue. If you experience any of these symptoms, it is important to see a healthcare provider for a proper diagnosis.

Diagnostic tests and Procedures

There are several diagnostic tests and procedures that can be used to diagnose breast cancer. These may include:

1.Mammography: This is a type of x-ray that is used to visualize the breast tissue. It can be used to detect breast cancer early, before it can be felt by hand.

2.Ultrasound: This test uses sound waves to create an image of the breast tissue. It can be used to determine whether a breast lump is a solid mass or a fluid-filled cyst.

3.Biopsy: A biopsy involves removing a sample of breast tissue to be examined under a microscope. There are several different types of biopsies that can be performed, including fine needle aspiration (FNA) biopsy, core needle biopsy, and surgical biopsy.

Staging: Once a diagnosis of breast cancer has been made, the next step is to determine the stage of the cancer. This involves determining the size of the tumor, whether it has spread to the lymph nodes or other parts of the body, and the overall health of the patient.

Other tests: Other tests that may be used in the diagnosis and staging of breast cancer include blood tests, imaging tests such as computerized tomography (CT) scans or positron emission tomography (PET) scans, and bone scans.

Types of Breast Cancer

1.Ductal carcinoma in situ (DCIS):

Ductal carcinoma in situ (DCIS) is a type of non-invasive(does not spread to other parts of the breast) breast cancer. It means that the cancer cells are confined to the milk ducts of the breast and have not spread to other parts of the body or invade nearby tissue. DCIS is considered to be an early stage of breast cancer and, if detected and treated promptly, has a high cure rate.

DCIS is typically found through a mammogram, a diagnostic test that uses low-dose X-rays to create images of the breast. It can also be detected during a breast biopsy, a procedure in which a sample of breast tissue is removed and examined under a microscope.

The most common symptoms of DCIS are a breast lump or thickening, and changes in the size or shape of the breast. However, many people with DCIS do not experience any symptoms, and the condition is often found during routine mammography.

Treatment options for DCIS include surgery (such as a lumpectomy or mastectomy), radiation therapy, and hormone therapy. The specific treatment plan will depend on the size and location of the DCIS, as well as the patient's overall health and preferences.

It is important to note that DCIS is not the same as invasive breast cancer, which means that the cancer cells have spread beyond the milk ducts into surrounding breast tissue. However, people with DCIS are at an increased risk of developing invasive breast cancer in the future, so it is important to follow up with regular

mammograms and other breast cancer screening tests as recommended by a healthcare provider.

2.Invasive ductal carcinoma:

Invasive ductal carcinoma (IDC) is a type of breast cancer that starts in the cells of the ducts (small tubes that carry milk to the nipple) and spreads beyond the ducts into the surrounding breast tissue. It is the most common type of breast cancer, accounting for about 80% of all cases.

IDC can occur at any age, but it is more common in women over 50. It can present as a lump or mass in the breast that can be felt during a self-examination or a clinical breast exam. Other symptoms may include a change in the size or shape of the breast, skin changes (such as dimpling or redness), nipple discharge, or changes in the way the nipple looks.

IDC is typically diagnosed through a combination of tests, including a physical exam, mammogram, ultrasound, and biopsy. The treatment for IDC depends on the stage of the cancer and may include surgery (such as a lumpectomy or mastectomy), radiation therapy, chemotherapy, and/or hormone therapy.

It is important for women to be aware of their breast health and to perform regular self-examinations and get regular mammograms as recommended by their healthcare provider. Early detection and treatment can greatly improve the chances of a successful outcome.

3.Invasive lobular carcinoma:

Invasive lobular carcinoma (ILC) is a type of breast cancer that begins in the lobules of the breast, which are the milk-producing glands. It is a less common type of breast cancer compared to invasive ductal carcinoma, which begins in the ducts of the breast.

Symptoms of ILC may include a breast lump, changes in the shape or size of the breast, and changes in the texture of the skin on the breast. However, many people with ILC do not experience any symptoms at all.

Diagnosis of ILC typically involves a combination of physical examination, mammography, ultrasound, and biopsy. If the cancer has spread beyond the breast, additional tests such as CT scans and bone scans may be needed to determine the extent of the disease.

Treatment for ILC may include surgery, chemotherapy, radiation therapy, and hormone therapy. The specific treatment plan will depend on the stage and characteristics of the cancer, as well as the overall health and preferences of the patient.

It is important for people with ILC to receive regular follow-up care after treatment to monitor for any recurrence of the cancer. This may include regular mammograms, physical exams, and other tests as needed.

Overall, the prognosis for ILC is generally good with appropriate treatment. However, it is important to catch the cancer early and seek treatment as soon as possible to increase the chances of a successful outcome.

Other types of breast cancer

There are several types of breast cancer, the most common of which is ductal carcinoma, which starts in the cells that line the milk ducts. Other types of breast cancer include:

I.Lobular carcinoma: This type of breast cancer starts in the lobules, which are the milk-producing glands in the breast.

II.Inflammatory breast cancer: This is a rare and aggressive form of breast cancer that affects the lymph vessels in the skin of the breast. It can cause the breast to become red, swollen, and warm to the touch.

III.Paget's disease of the breast: This type of breast cancer affects the skin of the nipple and the area surrounding it. It can cause the skin to become red, scaly, and crusty.

IV.Mucinous carcinoma: This type of breast cancer produces a large amount of mucus, which can cause the breast to feel like it is filled with fluid.

V.Medullary carcinoma: This is a rare type of breast cancer that tends to grow slowly and is usually found in women under the age of 50.

VI.Metaplastic carcinoma: This is a rare and aggressive form of breast cancer that can appear in any part of the breast and can have different types of cells, such as squamous cells or bone cells.

It's important to note that the type of breast cancer and its treatment will depend on the specific characteristics of the cancer cells and the stage of the cancer. It's important to consult with a healthcare provider for a proper diagnosis and treatment plan.

Staging and Grading Systems

Staging System

The staging of breast cancer refers to the extent to which the cancer has spread in the body. It is an important factor in determining the treatment options and the prognosis (outlook) for the patient. The most widely used staging system for breast cancer is the TNM system, developed by the American Joint Committee on Cancer (AJCC).

In the TNM system, the T refers to the size and extent of the primary tumor, the N refers to the presence and extent of lymph node involvement, and the M refers to the presence of distant metastasis (spread of the cancer to other parts of the body). Each of these factors is assigned a number or letter, and the stage of the cancer is determined by combining these values.

For example, a stage II breast cancer would be designated as T2 N1 M0, indicating that the primary tumor is larger than 2 cm but not larger than 5 cm, there is involvement of 1 to 3 lymph nodes, and there is no evidence of distant metastasis. A stage IV breast cancer, on the other hand, would be designated as any T, any N, and M1, indicating that the cancer has spread to distant parts of the body.

The stages of breast cancer are generally divided into five categories:

Stage 0: Also called noninvasive or in situ breast cancer, this stage refers to cancer that is confined to the breast tissue and has not spread to other parts of the body.

Stage I: At this stage, the cancer is still confined to the breast and is relatively small. It may have spread to the lymph nodes in the armpit (axillary lymph nodes), but there is no evidence of metastasis.

Stage II: At this stage, the cancer may be larger and may have spread to the lymph nodes in the armpit, but there is still no evidence of metastasis.

Stage III: At this stage, the cancer has spread beyond the breast and lymph nodes in the armpit, but is still confined to the chest. It may have spread to the lymph nodes in the chest or to the skin of the breast.

Stage IV: This is the most advanced stage of breast cancer, and it refers to cancer that has spread to other parts of the body, such as the bones, liver, or lungs.

It is important to note that the TNM staging system is just one way to stage breast cancer, and different staging systems may be used in different countries or by different cancer organizations. Additionally, the stage of a breast cancer can change over time as the cancer grows or spreads, and it is important for patients to have regular follow-up care to monitor the progression of the cancer.

Grading System

Breast cancer is graded based on how abnormal the cancer cells look under a microscope and how likely the cancer is to grow and spread. The grading system helps doctors predict the behavior of the cancer and determine the most appropriate treatment.

There are several different grading systems used to grade breast cancer, but the most widely used is the Nottingham grading system. This system uses three factors to grade the cancer: the appearance of the cancer cells under the microscope (histologic grade), the proliferation rate of the cancer cells (mitotic grade), and the presence of certain markers on the cancer cells (marker grade).

The histologic grade is based on the appearance of the cancer cells under the microscope. It takes into account the size and shape of the cells, as well as the presence of certain features that are associated with more aggressive cancer, such as nuclear pleomorphism (abnormal cell shape and size) and necrosis (cell death).

The mitotic grade is based on the proliferation rate of the cancer cells. It measures the number of cells that are actively dividing (mitosis) in the cancer tissue. A higher mitotic grade indicates a higher proliferation rate, which is associated with a more aggressive cancer.

The marker grade is based on the presence of certain markers on the cancer cells, such as estrogen and progesterone receptors and human epidermal growth factor receptor 2 (HER2). These markers can help predict the likelihood of the cancer responding to certain types of treatment.

The three grades are combined to give the overall cancer grade, which is assigned a number from 1 to 3. Grade 1 tumors are considered low-grade, while grade 3 tumors are considered high-grade. Low-grade tumors tend to grow and spread more slowly than high-grade tumors, and they are generally associated with a better prognosis.

It's important to note that the grade of a breast cancer does not determine the stage of the cancer. The stage of breast cancer refers to the extent of the cancer in the body and is determined by

factors such as the size of the tumor, whether the cancer has spread to the lymph nodes, and whether it has spread to other parts of the body.

Treatment Options

Breast cancer treatment typically involves a combination of surgery, chemotherapy, radiation therapy, and hormone therapy. The specific treatment options recommended for an individual with breast cancer will depend on the type and stage of the cancer, as well as the person's age, overall health, and preferences.

1.Surgery: Surgery is often the first line of treatment for breast cancer. There are several types of surgery that may be used to treat breast cancer, including:

I.Lumpectomy: This surgery involves removing the cancerous tumor and a small amount of surrounding healthy tissue.

II.Mastectomy: This surgery involves removing the entire breast. There are several types of mastectomy, including partial mastectomy, total mastectomy, and radical mastectomy.

III.Lymph node surgery: If the cancer has spread to the lymph nodes, surgery may be performed to remove the affected lymph nodes.

2.Chemotherapy: Chemotherapy is a type of treatment that uses drugs to kill cancer cells. It may be used before or after surgery to shrink the tumor and kill any remaining cancer cells, or it may be used as a standalone treatment for advanced breast cancer.

3.Radiation therapy: Radiation therapy uses high-energy beams, such as x-rays, to kill cancer cells. It may be used after surgery to destroy any remaining cancer cells and reduce the risk of the cancer coming back.

4.Hormone therapy: Hormone therapy is a type of treatment that targets hormones that can fuel the growth of certain types of breast cancer. It may be used to treat hormone receptor-positive breast cancer, which means that the cancer cells have receptors for hormones such as estrogen and progesterone. Hormone therapy may involve drugs that block the production or action of hormones, or it may involve surgery to remove the hormone-producing organs, such as the ovaries or adrenal glands.

5.Targeted therapy: This treatment targets specific proteins or genetic changes in cancer cells. It may be used in combination with other treatments, such as chemotherapy, to help kill cancer cells.

It's important to note that the treatment of breast cancer is constantly evolving, and new therapies are being developed all the time. It's important for individuals with breast cancer to work closely with their healthcare team to determine the most appropriate treatment plan for their specific situation.

Living With Breast Cancer

Coping with a Cancer Diagnosis

A breast cancer diagnosis can be a traumatic and overwhelming experience for anyone. It can be difficult to cope with the emotional, physical, and logistical challenges that come with it. However, there are several strategies you can use to help manage your emotions and support yourself during this time.

1.Seek support: It's important to have a strong support system during this time. This could include friends, family, a support group, or a therapist. It can be helpful to talk about your feelings and concerns with someone who understands what you're going through.

2.Take care of your physical health: It's important to take care of your physical health during treatment. This may include getting enough rest, eating well, and staying active. It's also important to follow your treatment plan as prescribed by your healthcare team.

3.Find ways to manage stress: Stress can make it harder to cope with a cancer diagnosis. Find ways to manage stress, such as through relaxation techniques, exercise, or hobbies. It can also be helpful to set limits on how much you take on and to ask for help when you need it.

4.Practice self-care: Taking care of yourself is crucial during this time. This could include activities like getting enough sleep, eating well, and finding time for relaxation and self-care.

5.Seek out reliable information: It can be helpful to learn as much as you can about your diagnosis and treatment options. However, it's important to get information from reliable sources, such as your healthcare team or reputable websites.

6.Practice mindfulness: Focusing on the present moment can help you cope with stress and anxiety. Consider trying mindfulness techniques such as deep breathing, meditation, or yoga.

Remember that everyone copes with a cancer diagnosis differently. It's important to find what works for you and to be patient with yourself as you navigate this difficult time.

Support for breast cancer survivors

Breast cancer survivors may face a variety of physical, emotional, and social challenges following treatment. It is important for breast cancer survivors to have access to support and resources to help them navigate these challenges and improve their quality of life.

One important source of support for breast cancer survivors is a healthcare team that includes medical professionals such as oncologists, surgeons, and primary care doctors, as well as mental health professionals, physical therapists, and other specialists. These professionals can provide medical care, counseling, and support to help survivors manage the physical and emotional effects of cancer and its treatment.

Support groups, both in-person and online, can also be a valuable resource for breast cancer survivors. These groups provide a safe and supportive environment for survivors to share their experiences and concerns with others who have gone through similar experiences. Support groups can also provide information and resources to help survivors cope with cancer-related challenges.

There are also many organizations and foundations that provide support for breast cancer survivors, including financial assistance, transportation to appointments, and access to resources such as wigs and prosthetics. These organizations may also offer educational programs and events, such as seminars and workshops, to help survivors learn more about their cancer and treatment options.

It is important for breast cancer survivors to prioritize their own self-care, which may include activities such as exercising, eating a healthy diet, and seeking support from loved ones and professionals. By taking care of themselves and accessing the support and resources that are available, breast cancer survivors can improve their quality of life and overall well-being.

Prevention and Screening for Breast Cancer

Risk Reduction Strategies

There are several strategies that can help reduce the risk of developing breast cancer:

1.Maintain a healthy weight: Being overweight or obese has been linked to an increased risk of breast cancer, particularly after menopause. Maintaining a healthy weight through a balanced diet and regular physical activity can help lower the risk.

2.Limit alcohol consumption: Studies have shown that the more alcohol a person consumes, the higher their risk of breast cancer. Limiting alcohol intake to no more than one drink per day can help reduce this risk.

3.Avoid or limit hormone therapy: Hormone therapy, particularly with combined estrogen and progestin, has been linked to an increased risk of breast cancer. If hormone therapy is necessary, the lowest effective dose should be used for the shortest possible time.

4.Breastfeed, if possible: Breastfeeding has been linked to a lower risk of breast cancer, particularly for women who breastfeed for one year or more.

5.Get regular screenings: Regular mammograms and clinical breast exams can help detect breast cancer early, when it is most treatable. It is recommended that women over the age of 50 get a mammogram every two years, and women at higher risk should talk to their healthcare provider about more frequent screenings.

6.Consider prophylactic surgery: For women who have a high risk of breast cancer due to genetic mutations or other factors, prophylactic surgery to remove the breasts or ovaries may be an option to consider. This should be carefully discussed with a healthcare provider.

7.Practice healthy lifestyle habits: Engaging in regular physical activity, eating a healthy diet rich in fruits and vegetables, and avoiding tobacco can all help reduce the risk of breast cancer.

Screening Tests

There are several screening tests that can be used to detect breast cancer, including:

1.Mammography: This is an X-ray of the breast tissue that can detect abnormalities that may indicate cancer. It is usually recommended for women over the age of 50, but may be recommended earlier for women with a family history of breast cancer or other risk factors.

2.Breast ultrasound: This test uses sound waves to create an image of the breast tissue. It is often used in conjunction with mammography to help determine the nature of an abnormal finding.

3.Breast Magnetic Resonance Imaging (MRI): This test uses magnetic fields and radio waves to create detailed images of the breast tissue. It is often used in women with a high risk of breast cancer or in women who have had breast cancer before.

4.Physical examination: During a physical examination, a healthcare provider will feel the breast tissue for lumps or abnormalities. This is usually done in conjunction with other screening tests.

5.Breast self-examination: Women are encouraged to perform breast self-examinations on a regular basis to check for any changes in their breast tissue. It is important to talk to a healthcare provider about how to properly perform a breast self-examination.

It is important to talk to a healthcare provider about the appropriate breast cancer screening tests based on an individual's age, risk factors, and personal preferences. The likelihood of successful therapy is significantly increased when breast cancer is detected at an earlier stage.

Conclusion and Future Directions

Advances in Breast Cancer Research

Cancer of the breast is the most prevalent form of the disease in women around the world and the second most prevalent form of cancer overall. In recent years, there have been significant advances in the field of breast cancer research, which have led to improved diagnosis, treatment, and survival rates for patients.

One area of research that has made significant progress is in the early detection of breast cancer. Advances in mammography and other imaging techniques, such as breast MRI and breast ultrasound, have made it possible to detect breast cancer at an earlier stage, when it is more treatable. There have also been developments in the use of biomarkers, such as the protein HER2, to help identify patients who may benefit from targeted therapies.

Another important area of breast cancer research has focused on the development of new treatments. There have been numerous advances in chemotherapy and hormonal therapies, including the use of targeted therapies such as trastuzumab (Herceptin) and lapatinib (Tykerb), which are specifically designed to attack cancer cells that overexpress the HER2 protein. There have also been developments in the use of immunotherapies, which harness the power of the immune system to fight cancer.

In addition to these advances, there has also been a greater emphasis on personalized medicine in breast cancer treatment. This involves using genetic testing to identify specific mutations and other characteristics of a patient's cancer, and then tailoring treatment to the individual based on these findings.

Overall, the progress made in breast cancer research over the past few decades has led to significant improvements in the diagnosis and treatment of this disease, and has helped to increase survival rates for patients. While there is still much work to be done, these advances offer hope for the future of breast cancer treatment and the possibility of even more effective therapies.

Ongoing Efforts to Improve Diagnosis and Treatment

There are ongoing efforts in the medical field to improve diagnosis and treatment of various diseases and conditions. Some of these efforts include:

1.Development of new diagnostic tools: Researchers are constantly working on developing new and more accurate diagnostic tools, such as blood tests, imaging techniques, and biomarkers. These tools can help doctors identify diseases and conditions earlier and more accurately, leading to earlier and more effective treatment.

2.Personalized medicine: Personalized medicine involves tailoring treatment to an individual's specific needs and characteristics, such as their genetic makeup or risk factors for certain conditions. By taking a more personalized approach to treatment, doctors can more effectively target the root cause of a patient's condition and offer more effective therapies.

3.Use of technology: Many healthcare providers are adopting the use of technology to improve diagnosis and treatment. For example, electronic health records (EHRs) can help doctors track a patient's medical history and make more informed treatment decisions. Telemedicine, which allows patients to consult with healthcare providers remotely, is also becoming increasingly common and can help improve access to care in underserved areas.

4.Clinical trials: Clinical trials are research studies that involve testing new treatments, drugs, or diagnostic tools in humans to determine their effectiveness and safety. These trials help researchers understand how different treatments work and can ultimately lead to the development of new and improved treatments.

Overall, these efforts are helping to improve the accuracy and effectiveness of diagnosis and treatment, leading to better outcomes for patients.

www.ingramcontent.com/pod-product-compliance
Lightning Source LLC
Chambersburg PA
CBHW071553260726
48653CB00007BA/3034